Cancer Survival Guide

Understanding and Coping with the Disease

Phillip J. Richmond

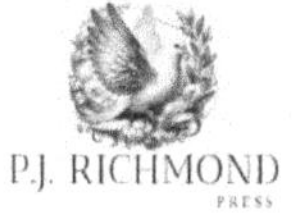

P.J. RICHMOND
PRESS

Dedication

Dedicated to all those touched by cancer—may this guide be a beacon of knowledge, support, and hope on your journey toward understanding, coping, and ultimately thriving in the face of adversity.

Also By Phillip J. Richmond

Contents

Introduction

Cancer is not just a disease; it's a journey that no one embarks on willingly. It's a path fraught with uncertainty, challenges, and profound questions about life, survival, and the very essence of what it means to be human. This book is a beacon of knowledge and hope for those who find themselves on this unexpected voyage. Cancer begins as a whisper in the body, a subtle shift in the way cells grow and divide. It's a complex array of diseases, each with its unique signature and impact on the body. Understanding cancer is akin to understanding a language foreign to our senses – it requires patience, attention, and a willingness to learn about the biological intricacies that define it.

At its core, cancer is a rebellion within the body's cellular community, where cells that once contributed to the body's harmony begin to divide without order or control. These rogue cells can invade other tissues and spread to different parts of the body, a process known as metastasis. The reasons behind this cellular insurrection are varied and complex, involving genetic, environmental, and lifestyle factors.

The Purpose of This Guide

This guide serves as a compass for navigating the tumultuous waters of a cancer diagnosis. It's crafted not only to educate but also to empower and inspire. The purpose of this guide is threefold:

1. To demystify the scientific jargon and present the facts about cancer in a clear, understandable manner.

2. To provide practical advice on coping with the physical and emotional toll of the disease.

3. To offer a source of solace and strength, reminding readers that they are not alone in this fight.

How to Use This Book

This book is structured to be your ally, whether you're a patient, a caregiver, or a concerned loved one. It's designed to be read in sequence or to be dipped into as needed, with each chapter addressing a specific aspect of the cancer experience.

- Start with the chapters on understanding cancer to build a solid foundation of knowledge.

- Proceed to the sections on treatment options and coping strategies to arm yourself with practical tools.

- Explore the personal stories and insights to find comfort and camaraderie.

In the pages that follow, you'll find a blend of scientific explanation, practical advice, and heartfelt storytelling. This book is a testament to the resilience of the human spirit and a guidebook for the journey ahead.

Chapter 1: What is Cancer?

Cancer, the word itself carries a weight that can silence rooms and halt the very flow of life. It's a diagnosis that no one wants to hear, yet it's one that millions of people must confront each year. But what exactly is cancer? This chapter will take you through the biological labyrinth of cancer, unraveling its complexities and demystifying its nature. At its most fundamental level, cancer is a disease of the cells. Our bodies are made up of trillions of cells, grouped into organs and tissues that perform specific functions. These cells have a life cycle: they are born, they grow, they divide, and when their time comes, they die. This cycle is tightly regulated by our DNA, the blueprint of life.

However, when this process goes awry, and cells begin to grow and divide uncontrollably, cancer can develop. These abnormal cells can form masses called tumors, which can be benign (non-cancerous) or malignant (cancerous). Malignant tumors can invade nearby tissues and spread to other parts of the body, a process known as metastasis. Cancer is often described as a genetic disease, but this doesn't mean it's always inherited. It's a disease of genes—the DNA in our cells—which can become damaged or mutated over time. These mutations can be the result of environmental exposures, such as tobacco smoke or ultraviolet rays, or they can occur randomly as cells divide. Some people inherit mutations from their parents that increase their risk of certain cancers. However, most cancers are the result of mutations that happen during a person's lifetime. These acquired mutations are the most common cause of cancer.

There are over 100 different types of cancer, and each is classified by the type of cell that is initially affected. Cancer harms the body when altered cells divide uncontrollably to form lumps or masses of tissue called tumors (except in the case of leukemia where cancer prohibits normal blood function by abnormal cell division in the bloodstream). Some cancers may eventually spread into other tissues, a process known as metastasis. The most common types of cancer in adults are breast, prostate, lung, and colorectal cancer. In children, the most common types are leukemia, brain tumors, and lymphoma.

Understanding cancer is the first step in the battle against it. This chapter has provided a glimpse into the intricate world of cancer biology, laying the groundwork for the subsequent chapters that will delve into diagnosis, treatment, and living with cancer. As we turn the page, we carry with us the knowledge that while cancer is indeed a formidable foe, it is one that we are learning more about every day, and one that we are increasingly equipped to fight against.

Chapter 2: Types of Cancer

Cancer's complexity is reflected in the diversity of its types. Broadly categorized by the origin of the malignant cells, cancers are classified into several main groups:

Carcinomas

Originating from epithelial cells, carcinomas are the most common type of cancer. They form in the skin or tissues lining the organs and glands. Subtypes include:

- **Adenocarcinoma**: Arising from mucus-secreting glands.
- **Basal cell carcinoma**: Developing in the basal cells of the skin.
- **Squamous cell carcinoma**: Stemming from the flat cells on the surface of the skin or lining of organs.

Sarcomas

These cancers originate from connective tissues such as bone, cartilage, and fat. Sarcomas are relatively rare and include:

- **Osteosarcoma**: Bone cancer typically found in children and young adults.
- **Liposarcoma**: Cancer of fat cells.
- **Chondrosarcoma**: Cancer of cartilage cells.

Leukemias

Leukemias are cancers of the blood-forming tissues, including the bone marrow. They do not form solid tumors but result in an overproduction of abnormal white blood cells. Types include:

- **Acute lymphoblastic leukemia (ALL)**: Most common in children.
- **Chronic lymphocytic leukemia (CLL)**: Typically affects adults over 55.
- **Acute myeloid leukemia (AML)**: Common in adults.
- **Chronic myeloid leukemia (CML)**: Mainly affects adults.

Lymphomas

Lymphomas start in the lymphatic system, which is part of the immune system. They are categorized into:

- **Hodgkin lymphoma**: Characterized by the presence of Reed-Sternberg cells.
- **Non-Hodgkin lymphoma**: A diverse group of blood cancers that includes many subtypes.

Brain and Spinal Cord Tumors

These tumors are named based on the type of cell they originate from and where they are located in the brain or spinal cord. Examples include:

- **Gliomas**: Arising from glial cells.
- **Meningiomas**: Originating from the meninges, the membranes that surround the brain and spinal cord.

The impact of cancer extends beyond the physical manifestations of the disease. It affects the emotional and psychological well-being of patients and their families. Coping with the diagnosis requires resilience and support, as well as a thorough understanding of the disease and its potential treatments. Treatment for cancer is as diverse as the disease itself, often involving a combination of surgery, chemotherapy, radiation therapy, and newer targeted therapies. The choice of treatment depends on the type and stage of cancer, as well as the patient's overall health and preferences.

Cancer is not a single disease but a collection of related diseases that can affect any part of the body. Understanding the types of cancer is crucial for effective treatment and coping strategies. As research advances, new therapies continue to emerge, offering hope and improved outcomes for patients worldwide.

Chapter 3: Causes and Risk Factors

Understanding the causes and risk factors associated with cancer is paramount in the journey toward prevention, early detection, and effective treatment. While the word "cancer" encompasses a diverse array of diseases, each with its own unique characteristics and triggers, there are overarching themes and commonalities that can shed light on how cancer develops and progresses within the human body.

1. Genetic Factors: A family history of certain cancers can be a sign of a possible inherited cancer syndrome. Genetic mutations can increase the risk of developing certain cancers. For example, the BRCA1 and BRCA2 genes are associated with an increased risk of breast and ovarian cancers.

2. Lifestyle Factors: Certain behaviors and habits can increase the risk of developing cancer. These include smoking, excessive alcohol consumption, and exposure to ultraviolet (UV) radiation from the sun or tanning bed.

3. Environmental Factors: Exposure to chemicals or other substances in the environment can also contribute to the risk of cancer. For example, asbestos exposure is linked to an increased risk of lung cancer, and exposure to certain pesticides can increase the risk of leukemia.

4. Age: The risk of developing cancer increases with age, as the body's cells accumulate mutations over time.

5. Diet and Nutrition: A diet low in fruits and vegetables and high in processed foods and red meat has been associated with an increased risk of certain cancers, such as colorectal cancer.

6. Infections: Certain viruses and bacteria can cause cancer. For example, the human papillomavirus (HPV) is linked to cervical, vaginal, and anal cancers, and hepatitis B and C viruses are associated with liver cancer.

7. Physical Activity and Obesity: Lack of physical activity and obesity have been linked to an increased risk of several types of cancer, including breast, colorectal, and endometrial cancers.

8. Stress and Emotional Well-Being: High levels of stress and poor emotional well-being have been associated with an increased risk of certain cancers, such as breast cancer.

9. Hormonal Factors: Hormonal imbalances, such as those caused by hormone replacement therapy, can increase the risk of certain cancers, such as breast cancer.

10. Inherited Genetic Syndromes: Certain inherited genetic syndromes, such as Lynch syndrome and Li-Fraumeni syndrome, can increase the risk of developing certain cancers.

It is essential to understand that not all cancers can be prevented, and not everyone who is exposed to these risk factors will develop cancer. However, by limiting exposure to avoidable risk factors and maintaining a healthy lifestyle, individuals can lower their risk of developing certain cancers. Early detection and regular screenings are also crucial for identifying and treating cancer at an early stage, when it is more treatable.

Chapter 4: Signs and Symptoms

Recognizing the signs and symptoms of cancer is the first step toward early detection, prompt intervention, and improved outcomes. While the manifestations of cancer can vary widely depending on the type, location, and stage of the disease, there are certain warning signs and common symptoms that individuals should be vigilant about.

1. **Unexplained Weight Loss**: Sudden and unexplained weight loss, especially when not accompanied by changes in diet or physical activity, can be a red flag for various types of cancer. Cancer cells consume energy and nutrients at an accelerated rate, leading to metabolic changes that result in unintentional weight loss. While occasional fluctuations in weight are normal, persistent and unexplained weight loss of 10 pounds or more should prompt further evaluation by a healthcare professional.

2. **Fatigue**: Cancer-related fatigue is a pervasive and debilitating symptom experienced by many cancer patients,

often described as an overwhelming sense of physical, emotional, and mental exhaustion that does not improve with rest. Fatigue may be caused by the cancer itself, as well as by cancer treatments such as chemotherapy, radiation therapy, and surgery. It is essential for patients to communicate their fatigue levels with their healthcare team, as interventions such as exercise, nutrition counseling, and medication management can help alleviate symptoms and improve quality of life.

3. Persistent Pain: Chronic or persistent pain that does not resolve with conventional treatments may be indicative of an underlying cancerous growth or tumor. Depending on the location and size of the tumor, pain may manifest as dull, achy discomfort or sharp, stabbing sensations. It is crucial for individuals to pay attention to any new or unusual pain symptoms, particularly if they persist for more than a few weeks, and to consult with a healthcare professional for further evaluation and management.

4. Changes in Bowel or Bladder Habits: Changes in bowel or bladder habits, such as persistent diarrhea, constipation, blood in the stool or urine, or urinary frequency and urgency, can be potential warning signs of colorectal, bladder, or prostate cancer. These symptoms may be indicative of underlying gastrointestinal or genitourinary malignancies and should not be ignored. Prompt evaluation by a healthcare provider, along with appropriate diagnostic tests such as colonoscopy, cystoscopy, or imaging studies, is essential for accurate diagnosis and treatment planning.

5. Persistent Cough or Hoarseness: A persistent cough, hoarseness, or wheezing that does not improve with conventional treatments may be indicative of lung cancer or other respiratory malignancies. While coughing is a common symptom of respiratory infections and allergies, persistent coughing accompanied by other worrisome symptoms such as chest pain, shortness of breath, or coughing up blood should prompt further investigation by a healthcare professional.

6. Changes in Skin: Changes in the appearance of the skin, such as new or changing moles, sores that do not heal, or unusual growths, should be evaluated by a dermatologist or healthcare provider. Skin cancers such as melanoma, basal cell carcinoma, and squamous cell carcinoma often present as changes in the size, shape, color, or texture of existing moles or lesions. Early detection and treatment of skin cancer are crucial for preventing metastasis and improving outcomes.

7. Difficulty Swallowing or Persistent Indigestion: Difficulty swallowing, persistent indigestion, or discomfort in the chest or throat may be indicative of esophageal, gastric, or gastrointestinal cancers. These symptoms may be accompanied by other signs such as unexplained weight loss, nausea, vomiting, or regurgitation of food. Individuals experiencing persistent gastrointestinal symptoms should seek evaluation by a healthcare professional, who may recommend diagnostic tests such as endoscopy or imaging studies to assess the underlying cause.

8. Changes in Breast Tissue: Changes in the breast tissue, including lumps, thickening, dimpling, or changes in size or shape, should be promptly evaluated by a healthcare provider. While many breast changes are benign, they can also be indicative of breast cancer, especially if accompanied by other symptoms such as nipple discharge, nipple inversion, or skin changes on the breast or nipple. Regular breast self-exams, clinical breast exams, and mammography are essential for early detection and treatment of breast cancer.

9. Neurological Symptoms: Neurological symptoms such as headaches, seizures, vision changes, numbness or weakness in the extremities, or difficulty speaking or understanding language can be indicative of brain or central nervous system tumors. While these symptoms can be caused by a variety of underlying conditions, persistent or progressive neurological symptoms should prompt further evaluation by a healthcare professional, who may recommend imaging studies such as MRI or CT scans to assess the presence of a brain tumor.

10. Unexplained Bleeding: Unexplained bleeding or bruising, such as blood in the stool, urine, or sputum, abnormal vaginal bleeding, or easy bruising without apparent cause, should be evaluated by a healthcare professional. These symptoms may be indicative of underlying hematological malignancies such as leukemia or lymphoma, as well as gastrointestinal, genitourinary, or gynecological cancers. Prompt evaluation and appropriate diagnostic testing are essential for accurate diagnosis and treatment planning.

In conclusion, being aware of the signs and symptoms associated with cancer empowers individuals to take proactive steps in advocating for their health and seeking timely medical attention when necessary. While many symptoms may be indicative of benign conditions or other non-cancerous causes, it is essential not to ignore persistent or worrisome symptoms and to consult with a healthcare professional for further evaluation and guidance. Early detection and intervention are critical in improving outcomes and maximizing quality of life for individuals affected by cancer.

Chapter 5: Diagnosis and Staging

An accurate diagnosis and detailed staging process are the first steps in the fight against cancer. This chapter focuses into the complex process of detecting cancer, identifying its extent and severity, and selecting the best course of therapy. Understanding the subtleties of cancer diagnosis and staging allows patients to confidently navigate the healthcare system, advocate for their needs, and make educated decisions regarding their care.

1. Clinical Evaluation: The diagnostic journey often begins with a thorough clinical evaluation by a healthcare provider, who takes a detailed medical history, performs a physical examination, and assesses presenting symptoms. During this initial assessment, the healthcare provider may inquire about risk factors, family history of cancer, lifestyle habits, and any concerning signs or symptoms that may warrant further investigation.

2. Diagnostic Imaging: Diagnostic imaging plays a crucial role in the detection, localization, and characterization of cancerous lesions within the body. Various imaging modalities such as X-rays, ultrasound, computed tomography (CT) scans, magnetic resonance imaging (MRI), and positron emission tomography (PET) scans may be utilized to visualize internal structures, assess tumor size and location, and evaluate for the presence of metastatic spread.

3. Biopsy: A biopsy involves the removal of a small sample of tissue or cells from a suspicious lesion or tumor for pathological examination under a microscope. Biopsies may be performed using minimally invasive techniques such as fine needle aspiration (FNA), core needle biopsy, or endoscopic biopsy, depending on the location and accessibility of the tumor. Pathological analysis of biopsy specimens enables clinicians to confirm the presence of cancer, characterize its histological subtype, and assess molecular biomarkers that may guide treatment decisions.

4. Laboratory Tests: Laboratory tests such as blood tests, urine tests, and tumor markers may provide valuable information about the presence of cancer, its biological behavior, and its response to treatment. Common tumor markers include prostate-specific antigen (PSA) for prostate cancer, carcinoembryonic antigen (CEA) for colorectal cancer, and CA-125 for ovarian cancer. While tumor markers are not definitive diagnostic tools on their own, they can complement other diagnostic modalities and help monitor disease progression over time.

5. Endoscopic Procedures: Endoscopic procedures such as colonoscopy, bronchoscopy, cystoscopy, and upper gastrointestinal endoscopy allow for direct visualization of internal organs and tissues, as well as the collection of biopsy samples for pathological analysis. Endoscopic examinations are instrumental in diagnosing cancers of the gastrointestinal tract, respiratory system, urinary tract, and other anatomical sites, enabling clinicians to assess tumor size, location, and extent of invasion.

6. Surgical Exploration: In some cases, surgical exploration may be necessary to obtain tissue samples for diagnostic purposes, particularly when other biopsy techniques are inconclusive or inaccessible. Surgical biopsies may be performed as open procedures or minimally invasive surgeries, depending on the location and size of the tumor and the overall health status of the patient. Surgical exploration allows for comprehensive tissue sampling and intraoperative assessment of tumor margins, lymph node involvement, and adjacent organ involvement.

7. Staging: Once a diagnosis of cancer has been established, the next step is to determine the stage of the disease, which describes the extent of tumor growth and spread within the body. Cancer staging is based on various factors, including tumor size, lymph node involvement, presence of metastases, and histological grade. The TNM (Tumor, Node, Metastasis) staging system is commonly used to classify cancer stages, with Stage 0 indicating in situ or localized disease and Stage IV indicating metastatic spread to distant organs.

8. Imaging Staging: Imaging studies such as CT scans, MRI scans, PET scans, and bone scans play a crucial role in staging cancer by providing detailed anatomical information about the extent and spread of the disease. These imaging modalities allow clinicians to visualize primary tumors, assess lymph node involvement, detect distant metastases, and evaluate the overall burden of disease within the body.

9. Pathological Staging: Pathological staging involves the examination of tumor tissue samples obtained from biopsies or surgical resections to assess the extent of tumor invasion, lymph node involvement, and presence of metastases. Pathological staging provides valuable information about the biological behavior of the cancer, its aggressiveness, and its potential response to treatment. Pathological staging is particularly important in guiding surgical management and adjuvant therapy decisions.

10. Multidisciplinary Consultation: Cancer diagnosis and staging often require a multidisciplinary approach involving collaboration among various healthcare professionals, including oncologists, surgeons, radiologists, pathologists, and other specialists. Multidisciplinary tumor boards or conferences bring together experts from different disciplines to review diagnostic findings, discuss treatment options, and formulate individualized care plans tailored to the unique needs of each patient.

The process of cancer diagnosis and staging is a complex and multifaceted journey that requires careful consideration of clinical, radiological, pathological, and molecular information. By leveraging a comprehensive array of diagnostic tools and expertise, healthcare providers can accurately assess the extent and severity of cancer, inform treatment decisions, and optimize outcomes for individuals affected by this disease. Empowering patients with knowledge about the diagnostic process and the importance of staging enables them to actively participate in their care and embark on the path toward cancer survival and resilience.

Chapter 6: Surgery

One of the cornerstones of a complete cancer treatment plan is surgery, which provides hope, healing, and the possibility of a cure. This chapter examines the wide range of surgical techniques used in cancer care, including reconstructive surgery, curative resections, and diagnostic biopsies. Knowing how surgery plays a part in cancer care enables patients to make knowledgeable decisions about their course of treatment and to face the challenges of surgical treatments with courage and resiliency.

1. Diagnostic Biopsy: A diagnostic biopsy is often the first step in confirming a suspected diagnosis of cancer, enabling clinicians to obtain tissue samples for pathological examination and molecular analysis. Biopsies may be performed using minimally invasive techniques such as fine needle aspiration (FNA), core needle biopsy, or endoscopic biopsy, depending on the location and accessibility of the tumor. The results of the biopsy inform subsequent treatment decisions and guide the selection of appropriate surgical interventions.

2. Curative Resection: Curative surgical resection involves the removal of the primary tumor and surrounding tissue with the goal of achieving complete eradication of cancerous cells. Depending on the type, location, and stage of the cancer, curative resections may be performed using open surgical techniques or minimally invasive approaches such as laparoscopy or robotic-assisted surgery. Curative resections are often complemented by adjuvant therapies such as chemotherapy or radiation therapy to target residual cancer cells and reduce the risk of recurrence.

3. Debulking Surgery: Debulking surgery is performed with the aim of reducing the size of a tumor or alleviating symptoms associated with tumor growth, particularly in cases where complete eradication of the cancer is not feasible. Debulking procedures may be employed as part of a multimodal treatment approach to improve the effectiveness of subsequent therapies such as chemotherapy or radiation therapy. Debulking surgery may be indicated in advanced or metastatic cancers to alleviate pain, improve quality of life, and prolong survival.

4. Lymph Node Dissection: Lymph node dissection, also known as lymphadenectomy, involves the surgical removal of regional lymph nodes to assess for the presence of cancer spread and to prevent further dissemination of the disease. Lymph node dissection is commonly performed in conjunction with primary tumor resection to accurately stage the cancer and guide adjuvant treatment decisions. Sentinel lymph node biopsy, a minimally invasive technique, may be utilized to identify and sample the first lymph nodes draining from the primary tumor site, reducing the extent of lymph node dissection while maintaining diagnostic accuracy.

5. Reconstructive Surgery: Reconstructive surgery plays a crucial role in restoring form and function following ablative procedures such as mastectomy, prostatectomy, or head and neck surgery. Reconstructive techniques may involve the use of autologous tissue flaps, tissue expanders, implants, or prosthetic devices to rebuild and reshape anatomical structures affected by cancer resection. Reconstructive surgery aims to enhance physical appearance, improve quality of life, and promote psychological well-being in cancer survivors.

6. Organ Preservation Surgery: Organ preservation surgery focuses on preserving vital organs and tissues while effectively treating cancer, particularly in cases where radical resection may result in significant functional impairment or loss of quality of life. Organ preservation techniques such as lumpectomy for breast cancer, sphincter-sparing surgery for rectal cancer, and larynx-preserving surgery for laryngeal cancer aim to achieve oncological control while preserving organ function and minimizing long-term morbidity.

7. Minimally Invasive Surgery: Minimally invasive surgical techniques such as laparoscopy and robotic-assisted surgery offer numerous advantages in the management of cancer, including reduced postoperative pain, shorter hospital stays, faster recovery times, and improved cosmetic outcomes. Minimally invasive approaches utilize small incisions and specialized instruments equipped with cameras and robotic arms to access and manipulate internal structures with precision and dexterity. Minimally invasive surgery may be employed for diagnostic biopsies, tumor resections, lymph node dissections, and reconstructive procedures across a wide range of cancer types.

8. Palliative Surgery: Palliative surgery focuses on relieving symptoms and improving quality of life in patients with advanced or metastatic cancer who may not be candidates for curative interventions. Palliative surgical procedures such as tumor debulking, stent placement, nerve blocks, and bypass surgeries aim to alleviate pain, alleviate obstruction or compression of vital organs, and manage complications associated with advanced cancer. Palliative surgery is often integrated into a comprehensive palliative care approach that addresses physical, emotional, and spiritual needs in patients with advanced illness.

9. Multidisciplinary Collaboration: Successful cancer surgery relies on a multidisciplinary approach involving collaboration among surgeons, oncologists, radiologists, pathologists, nurses, and other healthcare professionals. Multidisciplinary tumor boards or conferences bring together experts from different specialties to review diagnostic findings, discuss treatment options, and formulate individualized care plans tailored to the unique needs of each patient. Multidisciplinary collaboration ensures comprehensive assessment, personalized treatment strategies, and optimal outcomes for individuals undergoing cancer surgery.

10. Preoperative Preparation and Postoperative Care: Preoperative preparation and postoperative care are integral components of the surgical journey, aimed at optimizing patient outcomes, reducing complications, and promoting recovery. Preoperative preparation may involve medical optimization, nutritional support, psychological counseling, and patient education to address concerns and alleviate anxiety. Postoperative care encompasses pain management, wound care, physical therapy, and supportive services to facilitate healing, restore function, and enhance quality of life during the recovery period.

Surgery plays a central role in the multidisciplinary management of cancer, offering curative, palliative, and supportive interventions tailored to the unique needs of each patient. By understanding the diverse array of surgical options available, individuals can actively participate in their treatment journey, advocate for their needs, and embark on the path toward cancer survival and resilience. Empowering patients with knowledge about cancer surgery fosters confidence, hope, and a sense of agency in navigating the challenges of cancer diagnosis and treatment.

Chapter 7: Radiation Therapy

Radiation therapy is a key component in the full arsenal of cancer therapies, providing precise precision and substantial therapeutic advantages. In this chapter, we will look at the complexities of radiation therapy, its mechanisms of action, its various uses across cancer types, and its critical role in multidisciplinary cancer care. Understanding the theory and practice of radiation therapy enables people to make educated treatment decisions and negotiate the complexity of radiation oncology with confidence and tenacity.

1. Principles of Radiation Therapy: Radiation therapy harnesses high-energy beams of ionizing radiation to selectively target and destroy cancerous cells while sparing surrounding healthy tissues. Radiation works by damaging the DNA within cancer cells, disrupting their ability to divide and proliferate, ultimately leading to cell death. The goal of radiation therapy is to deliver a precise dose of radiation to the tumor while minimizing exposure to adjacent normal tissues, thereby maximizing therapeutic efficacy and minimizing treatment-related toxicity.

2. Types of Radiation Therapy: There are two primary types of radiation therapy: external beam radiation therapy (EBRT) and internal radiation therapy (brachytherapy). External beam radiation therapy delivers radiation from an external source outside the body, typically using a linear accelerator, to precisely target the tumor from multiple angles while minimizing radiation exposure to surrounding healthy tissues. Brachytherapy, on the other hand, involves the placement of radioactive sources directly within or adjacent to the tumor site, delivering a high dose of radiation locally while minimizing exposure to nearby structures.

3. Indications for Radiation Therapy: Radiation therapy may be employed as a primary treatment modality for certain localized cancers, as adjuvant therapy following surgical resection to reduce the risk of local recurrence, or as palliative therapy to alleviate symptoms and improve quality of life in patients with advanced or metastatic disease. Radiation therapy may be used alone or in combination with other treatment modalities such as surgery, chemotherapy, or targeted therapy, depending on the type, stage, and biological characteristics of the cancer.

4. Treatment Planning and Delivery: Radiation therapy treatment planning begins with a comprehensive evaluation of the patient's medical history, diagnostic imaging studies, and tumor characteristics to determine the optimal treatment approach. Advanced imaging techniques such as CT scans, MRI scans, and PET scans are utilized to precisely delineate the target volume and adjacent critical structures. Radiation oncologists collaborate with medical physicists, dosimetrists, and radiation therapists to develop customized treatment plans that deliver the prescribed dose of radiation while minimizing toxicity to healthy tissues.

5. Fractionation and Dose Optimization: Radiation therapy is typically delivered in multiple fractions over a period of several weeks to optimize tumor control while minimizing normal tissue toxicity. Fractionation allows for the delivery of higher cumulative doses of radiation to the tumor while allowing healthy tissues to repair and recover between treatments. Radiation dose and fractionation schedules are tailored to the specific characteristics of the tumor, including size, location, histology, and sensitivity to radiation.

6. Radiation Techniques and Modalities: Radiation therapy techniques continue to evolve, with advancements in technology enabling more precise and effective delivery of radiation to tumor targets. Modern radiation therapy modalities such as intensity-modulated radiation therapy (IMRT), stereotactic body radiation therapy (SBRT), proton therapy, and image-guided radiation therapy (IGRT) offer enhanced targeting accuracy, sparing of normal tissues, and reduced treatment-related toxicity compared to conventional radiation techniques.

7. Side Effects and Toxicities: While radiation therapy is a highly effective treatment modality, it can also cause side effects and toxicities, particularly when adjacent normal tissues are exposed to radiation. Common side effects of radiation therapy may include fatigue, skin irritation, hair loss, nausea, vomiting, and changes in bowel or bladder function. The severity and duration of side effects vary depending on factors such as the dose and volume of radiation, the location of the treatment site, and individual patient factors.

8. Management of Radiation-Induced Side Effects: Radiation oncologists work closely with supportive care providers to manage and mitigate treatment-related side effects and toxicities. Strategies for managing radiation-induced side effects may include supportive medications, topical treatments for skin irritation, dietary modifications, physical therapy, and psychosocial support services. Patient education and proactive symptom management are essential in optimizing treatment tolerance and quality of life during and after radiation therapy.

9. Long-Term Follow-Up and Survivorship Care: Following completion of radiation therapy, patients undergo regular follow-up appointments with their radiation oncologist to monitor treatment response, assess for recurrence or late effects, and provide ongoing supportive care. Long-term survivorship care focuses on addressing physical, emotional, and psychosocial needs in cancer survivors, promoting healthy lifestyle behaviors, and monitoring for late effects of radiation therapy such as secondary cancers, cardiac toxicity, or radiation-induced fibrosis.

10. Future Directions in Radiation Oncology: The field of radiation oncology continues to evolve rapidly, with ongoing research and technological innovations driving advancements in treatment delivery, imaging guidance, and targeted therapies. Emerging areas of interest in radiation oncology include immunotherapy combined with radiation, radiomics and artificial intelligence in treatment planning, and novel radiation sensitizers and radioprotectors to enhance therapeutic efficacy and minimize toxicity.

Radiation therapy plays a central role in the multidisciplinary management of cancer, offering precise and effective treatment options tailored to the unique needs of each patient. By understanding the principles, practice, and potential side effects of radiation therapy, individuals can make informed decisions about their treatment journey, advocate for their needs, and embark on the path toward cancer survival and resilience. Empowering patients with knowledge about radiation therapy fosters confidence, hope, and a sense of agency in navigating the challenges of cancer diagnosis and treatment.

Cancer cells can invade nearby tissues and organs, disrupting their normal function, and can also spread to other parts of the body through the bloodstream or lymphatic system, a process known as metastasis.

Chapter 8: Chemotherapy

In the vast landscape of cancer treatment, chemotherapy stands as one of the most formidable weapons against the disease. It is a multifaceted approach that involves the use of powerful drugs to target and destroy cancer cells, offering hope and healing to countless individuals battling cancer worldwide. However, the journey through chemotherapy is not without its challenges and uncertainties. Chemotherapy, often referred to simply as "chemo," works by interfering with the ability of cancer cells to grow and multiply. It employs a variety of drugs, each with its own mode of action, to attack cancer cells at different stages of their growth cycle. By targeting rapidly dividing cells, chemotherapy not only destroys cancerous cells but also may affect healthy cells in the body that divide rapidly, such as those in the bone marrow, digestive tract, and hair follicles.

The decision to undergo chemotherapy is a complex one that depends on several factors, including the type and stage of cancer, the overall health and preferences of the patient, and the goals of treatment. Chemotherapy may be used as a standalone treatment or in combination with surgery, radiation therapy, immunotherapy, or targeted therapy, forming part of a comprehensive treatment plan tailored to each individual's unique circumstances.

For many individuals, the prospect of undergoing chemotherapy can evoke feelings of fear, anxiety, and uncertainty. The treatment process can be physically demanding and emotionally draining, requiring a significant commitment of time, energy, and resources. However, with the support of a dedicated healthcare team and a strong support network, many patients navigate the challenges of chemotherapy with courage and resilience. The journey through chemotherapy typically begins with a thorough evaluation by a medical oncologist, who will recommend a specific chemotherapy regimen based on the type and stage of cancer, as well as other relevant factors. Chemotherapy drugs may be administered orally, intravenously, or through other routes, depending on the treatment protocol. Treatment schedules vary widely, with some regimens requiring daily, weekly, or monthly sessions over a period of several weeks or months.

While chemotherapy can be highly effective in fighting cancer, it can also cause a range of side effects that may vary in severity from mild to severe. Common side effects of chemotherapy may include:

- Nausea and vomiting.
- Fatigue.
- Hair loss.
- Loss of appetite.
- Changes in taste and smell.
- Mouth sores.
- Increased risk of infection due to suppressed immune function.
- Anemia.
- Peripheral neuropathy (numbness, tingling, or pain in the hands and feet).

Managing these side effects is an essential aspect of chemotherapy care, and patients are encouraged to communicate openly with their healthcare team about any symptoms or concerns they may experience. Supportive care measures, such as anti-nausea medications, pain management techniques, nutritional support, and emotional counseling, can help alleviate discomfort and improve quality of life during treatment.

Navigating the challenges of chemotherapy requires not only medical expertise but also emotional resilience and social support. Patients undergoing chemotherapy often find solace and strength in connecting with others who share similar experiences, whether through support groups, online communities, or one-on-one interactions with friends and family. In addition to seeking support from others, practicing self-care and prioritizing well-being are crucial aspects of coping with chemotherapy. Engaging in activities that bring joy and relaxation, such as gentle exercise, meditation, creative expression, and spending time outdoors, can help alleviate stress and promote a sense of balance and resilience.

As challenging as the journey through chemotherapy may be, it is important to remember that it is a temporary phase on the path to healing and recovery. With advances in medical research and supportive care, the landscape of cancer treatment continues to evolve, offering new hope and possibilities for those affected by the disease.

By approaching chemotherapy with courage, resilience, and a spirit of collaboration with healthcare professionals and loved ones, individuals can navigate the ups and downs of treatment with grace and dignity. Together, we can embrace the journey of cancer survival with hope, determination, and the unwavering belief in the power of the human spirit to overcome adversity and thrive in the face of challenges.

Common symptoms of cancer include persistent fatigue, unexplained weight loss, changes in bowel or bladder habits, persistent cough or hoarseness, and unusual bleeding or discharge.

Chapter 9: Immunotherapy

In the ongoing battle against cancer, the emergence of immunotherapy represents a revolutionary breakthrough in the field of oncology. Harnessing the power of the body's own immune system to recognize and attack cancer cells, immunotherapy offers new hope and promise to individuals facing a wide range of cancer types. At the heart of immunotherapy lies a simple yet profound concept: the human immune system possesses an innate ability to detect and destroy foreign invaders, including cancer cells. However, cancer cells often employ clever strategies to evade detection by the immune system, allowing them to proliferate unchecked and spread throughout the body. Immunotherapy works by reactivating and enhancing the body's immune response, enabling it to recognize and eliminate cancer cells more effectively.

There are several different approaches to immunotherapy, each targeting different aspects of the immune system's response to cancer. These include:

- **Checkpoint inhibitors**: Drugs that block the "checkpoints" on immune cells, preventing cancer cells from inhibiting the immune response and allowing the immune system to attack the tumor more effectively.

- **CAR-T cell therapy**: A personalized treatment approach in which a patient's own T cells are genetically engineered to recognize and kill cancer cells.

- **Monoclonal antibodies**: Laboratory-produced antibodies that target specific proteins on cancer cells, marking them for destruction by the immune system.

- **Cancer vaccines**: Vaccines designed to stimulate the immune system to recognize and attack cancer cells, either by targeting specific antigens present on the surface of cancer cells or by stimulating a more generalized immune response.

One of the most exciting aspects of immunotherapy is its potential for precision medicine, tailoring treatment approaches to the unique genetic makeup of each individual's cancer. By analyzing the genetic mutations and molecular characteristics of a patient's tumor, oncologists can identify specific targets for immunotherapy and design personalized treatment regimens that are more likely to be effective and less toxic than traditional chemotherapy or radiation therapy. Precision medicine approaches such as immunotherapy hold particular promise for individuals with advanced or treatment-resistant cancers, offering new hope where conventional treatments may have failed. Clinical trials evaluating the safety and efficacy of immunotherapy in a variety of cancer types continue to yield promising results, paving the way for the development of new and improved treatment options for patients around the world.

While immunotherapy represents a groundbreaking advancement in cancer treatment, it is not without its challenges and complexities. Like any medical intervention, immunotherapy can cause side effects ranging from mild to severe, depending on the specific treatment regimen and individual patient factors. Common side effects of immunotherapy may include:

- Fatigue.

- Skin rashes.

- Flu-like symptoms.

- Diarrhea or other gastrointestinal issues.

- Endocrine disorders.

- Immune-related adverse events, such as pneumonitis, hepatitis, or colitis.

Managing these side effects requires close collaboration between patients and their healthcare team, who will monitor for signs of toxicity and adjust treatment as needed to minimize discomfort and maximize effectiveness. In some cases, immunotherapy may be combined with other treatment modalities, such as chemotherapy, radiation therapy, or targeted therapy, to enhance its therapeutic effects and improve outcomes.

As we continue to unlock the mysteries of the immune system and harness its power to fight cancer, the future of immunotherapy shines brightly with promise and potential. With each new discovery and breakthrough, we move one step closer to a world where cancer is no longer a life-threatening diagnosis but a manageable chronic condition. For individuals facing cancer, immunotherapy offers not only a ray of hope but also a renewed sense of agency and empowerment in their journey toward healing and recovery. By embracing the possibilities of precision medicine, advocating for access to cutting-edge treatments, and fostering a spirit of resilience and optimism, we can collectively work towards a future where cancer survival is not only achievable but commonplace.

In the words of Dr. William Coley, a pioneering immunologist whose work laid the foundation for modern immunotherapy, "Cancer immunotherapy is not just a treatment option; it is a revolution in the making—a testament to the power of the human immune system to conquer disease and defy the odds." Together, let us march forward with courage, determination, and unwavering hope in the quest for a world free from the burden of cancer.

The treatment options for cancer depend on factors such as the type, stage, and location of the disease, and may include surgery, chemotherapy, radiation therapy, immunotherapy, targeted therapy, and hormone therapy.

Chapter 10: Targeted Therapy

In the ever-evolving landscape of cancer treatment, targeted therapy stands as a beacon of hope and innovation, offering precise and personalized approaches to combating the disease. Unlike traditional treatments such as chemotherapy, which often affect both cancerous and healthy cells, targeted therapy employs drugs or other substances that specifically target the molecular or genetic abnormalities driving cancer growth. At the core of targeted therapy lies a fundamental principle: the recognition that cancer is not a homogeneous disease but rather a collection of diverse and complex disorders characterized by unique molecular and genetic alterations. These alterations may arise from mutations, amplifications, or other changes in key genes or signaling pathways that drive abnormal cell growth and proliferation.

Targeted therapy aims to exploit these vulnerabilities by delivering drugs or other agents that specifically inhibit or block the activity of proteins, enzymes, or other molecules involved in cancer development and progression. By honing in on these molecular targets, targeted therapy offers the potential for more effective and less toxic treatment approaches, sparing healthy cells from the collateral damage often associated with traditional chemotherapy.

There are several different types of targeted therapy, each designed to address specific molecular targets or pathways implicated in cancer growth and survival. Some common types of targeted therapy include:

- **Small molecule inhibitors**: Drugs that interfere with the activity of specific proteins or enzymes involved in cancer cell signaling pathways, often by binding to them and blocking their function.

- **Monoclonal antibodies**: Laboratory-produced antibodies that target and bind to specific proteins on the surface of cancer cells, marking them for destruction by the immune system or inhibiting their growth and proliferation.

- **Signal transduction inhibitors**: Drugs that interfere with signaling pathways within cancer cells, disrupting the communication networks that drive abnormal cell growth and survival.

- **Angiogenesis inhibitors**: Drugs that inhibit the formation of new blood vessels, depriving tumors of the oxygen and nutrients they need to grow and spread.

Each type of targeted therapy may be used alone or in combination with other treatment modalities, such as chemotherapy, radiation therapy, or immunotherapy, depending on the specific characteristics of the cancer and the goals of treatment.

One of the most exciting aspects of targeted therapy is its potential for personalized medicine and precision oncology. By analyzing the molecular profile of a patient's tumor, oncologists can identify specific molecular targets or genetic alterations that are driving cancer growth and select targeted therapies that are most likely to be effective for that individual. This personalized approach allows for more tailored and effective treatment regimens, improving outcomes and minimizing side effects. Advances in genomic sequencing technologies have greatly expanded our understanding of the molecular underpinnings of cancer and the diversity of genetic alterations that contribute to its development and progression. As our knowledge continues to grow, so too does the arsenal of targeted therapies available to oncologists, offering new hope and possibilities for individuals facing a wide range of cancer types.

While targeted therapy holds great promise for the future of cancer treatment, it is not without its challenges and limitations. Like any medical intervention, targeted therapy can cause side effects ranging from mild to severe, depending on the specific drugs used and individual patient factors. Common side effects of targeted therapy may include:

- Skin rash or other dermatologic issues.
- Gastrointestinal disturbances.
- Fatigue.
- Elevated blood pressure or other cardiovascular effects.
- Liver toxicity.

- Immune-related adverse events, such as thyroid dysfunction or pneumonitis

Managing these side effects requires close collaboration between patients and their healthcare team, who will monitor for signs of toxicity and adjust treatment as needed to minimize discomfort and maximize effectiveness. In some cases, targeted therapy may be combined with other treatment modalities, such as chemotherapy or immunotherapy, to enhance its therapeutic effects and improve outcomes.

As we continue to unlock the molecular secrets of cancer and develop increasingly sophisticated targeted therapies, the future of cancer treatment shines brightly with hope and promise. With each new discovery and breakthrough, we move one step closer to a world where cancer is not only treatable but ultimately curable. For individuals facing cancer, targeted therapy offers not only a lifeline but also a renewed sense of optimism and empowerment in their journey toward healing and recovery. By embracing the possibilities of personalized medicine, advocating for access to cutting-edge treatments, and fostering a spirit of resilience and hope, we can collectively work towards a future where cancer survival is not only achievable but commonplace.

In the words of Dr. Siddhartha Mukherjee, author of "The Emperor of All Maladies: A Biography of Cancer," "Targeted therapy represents a triumph of precision and perseverance—a testament to the power of scientific inquiry and human ingenuity to conquer disease and defy the odds." Together, let us march forward with courage, determination, and unwavering hope in the quest for a world free from the burden of cancer.

Chapter 11: Alternative Treatments

In the journey through cancer, patients often find themselves exploring a multitude of treatment options beyond conventional medicine. Alternative treatments, ranging from herbal remedies to mind-body therapies, have gained attention for their potential to complement traditional approaches and improve overall well-being. However, it's crucial to approach these options with a critical mind, understanding their benefits, limitations, and potential risks. Holistic healing approaches aim to address the physical, emotional, and spiritual aspects of health. Practices such as acupuncture, massage therapy, and yoga have shown promise in alleviating treatment side effects, reducing stress, and enhancing quality of life for cancer patients. These modalities not only offer relaxation and pain relief but also promote a sense of empowerment and self-awareness.

Nutrition plays a crucial role in supporting the body's immune system and overall well-being during cancer treatment. Incorporating a balanced diet rich in fruits, vegetables, whole grains, and lean proteins can help maintain strength and vitality. Additionally, certain supplements, such as vitamin D, omega-3 fatty acids, and probiotics, may offer benefits in managing treatment side effects and boosting immune function. However, it's essential to consult with a healthcare professional before adding any supplements to your regimen, as they may interact with medications or exacerbate certain conditions.

Herbal remedies have been used for centuries in various cultures as natural treatments for a wide range of ailments, including cancer. Herbs like turmeric, ginger, and green tea contain potent antioxidants and anti-inflammatory compounds that may have cancer-fighting properties. While research on the efficacy of herbal remedies in cancer treatment is ongoing, some patients report experiencing symptom relief and improved quality of life through their use. It's important to approach herbal medicine with caution, ensuring proper dosage and discussing potential interactions with healthcare providers.

The mind-body connection plays a significant role in health and healing. Practices such as meditation, guided imagery, and hypnotherapy can help reduce stress, anxiety, and depression, thereby enhancing the body's ability to cope with cancer and its treatments. By cultivating mindfulness and relaxation techniques, individuals can tap into their innate resilience and foster a sense of inner peace amidst the challenges of cancer.

Complementary and integrative medicine combines conventional medical treatments with alternative therapies to provide comprehensive care for cancer patients. Integrative oncology programs offer a collaborative approach, incorporating evidence-based practices from both Western and Eastern traditions to address the physical, emotional, and spiritual needs of patients. These programs may include a combination of chemotherapy, radiation, surgery, nutritional counseling, acupuncture, massage therapy, and psychosocial support, tailored to each individual's unique circumstances and preferences.

While alternative treatments hold promise in supporting cancer care, it's essential to approach them with caution and skepticism. Not all alternative therapies are backed by scientific evidence, and some may even pose risks or interfere with conventional treatments. Before embarking on any alternative treatment regimen, it's crucial to consult with a knowledgeable healthcare provider who can provide guidance, monitor progress, and ensure safety.

Navigating the world of alternative treatments can be both empowering and daunting for cancer patients and their loved ones. By embracing a holistic approach to healing, incorporating evidence-based practices, and seeking guidance from healthcare professionals, individuals can complement their conventional treatment plans with alternative therapies that support their physical, emotional, and spiritual well-being. Ultimately, the journey through cancer is a deeply personal one, and finding the right combination of treatments and practices is key to thriving in the face of adversity.

Chapter 12: Nutrition and Cancer

Nutrition plays a pivotal role in the prevention, management, and overall well-being of individuals affected by cancer. As research continues to uncover the intricate relationship between diet and disease, it becomes increasingly evident that making informed dietary choices can significantly impact one's journey through cancer. A balanced diet rich in nutrient-dense foods serves as the cornerstone of cancer prevention and management. Fruits, vegetables, whole grains, lean proteins, and healthy fats provide essential vitamins, minerals, antioxidants, and phytochemicals that bolster the body's immune system, repair cellular damage, and inhibit the growth of cancerous cells. Incorporating a diverse array of colorful fruits and vegetables into meals not only adds flavor and texture but also delivers a potent dose of cancer-fighting compounds.

Antioxidants play a crucial role in neutralizing harmful free radicals, which can damage DNA and contribute to cancer development. Foods such as berries, nuts, seeds, leafy greens, and colorful fruits are rich sources of antioxidants, including vitamins A, C, and E, as well as selenium, zinc, and flavonoids. By including these antioxidant-rich foods in your diet, you can help protect cells from oxidative stress and reduce the risk of cancer progression.

Phytochemicals are bioactive compounds found in plants that possess potent anti-cancer properties. These include carotenoids, flavonoids, polyphenols, and glucosinolates, which exert various effects on cellular processes involved in cancer development and progression. Foods such as cruciferous vegetables (broccoli, cauliflower, Brussels sprouts), citrus fruits, tomatoes, soybeans, and green tea are abundant sources of phytochemicals that have been shown to inhibit tumor growth, promote apoptosis (cell death), and suppress inflammation.

In addition to vitamins, minerals, and phytochemicals, macronutrients such as carbohydrates, proteins, and fats play essential roles in supporting overall health and well-being during cancer treatment. Carbohydrates provide the body with energy and should be sourced from whole grains, fruits, and vegetables to ensure a steady supply of fiber, vitamins, and minerals. Proteins are crucial for tissue repair and immune function and should be obtained from lean sources such as poultry, fish, legumes, and tofu. Healthy fats, including omega-3 fatty acids found in fatty fish, nuts, and seeds, contribute to cardiovascular health and may help reduce inflammation associated with cancer.

During cancer treatment, nutritional needs may fluctuate depending on the type of treatment, side effects, and individual factors such as weight, age, and activity level. Some treatments, such as chemotherapy and radiation, can impact appetite, taste perception, and digestion, making it challenging to maintain adequate nutrition. In such cases, working with a registered dietitian or nutritionist who specializes in oncology can help develop personalized meal plans and strategies to optimize nutrient intake and manage treatment-related side effects.

After completing cancer treatment, survivors may face unique nutritional challenges as they transition into survivorship. Some individuals may experience long-term side effects such as gastrointestinal issues, neuropathy, or changes in taste and appetite, which can impact dietary choices and eating habits. It's essential for survivors to prioritize nutrition as part of their ongoing wellness plan, focusing on whole foods, regular physical activity, and maintaining a healthy weight to reduce the risk of cancer recurrence and promote overall longevity.

Nutrition serves as a powerful ally in the fight against cancer, offering a proactive approach to prevention, treatment support, and survivorship. By embracing a diet rich in nutrient-dense foods, antioxidants, and phytochemicals, individuals can nourish their bodies, strengthen their immune systems, and optimize their overall well-being throughout the cancer journey. As we continue to unravel the complex interplay between diet and disease, incorporating evidence-based nutrition strategies into comprehensive cancer care becomes increasingly vital for improving outcomes and enhancing quality of life.

Chapter 13: Managing Side Effects

Facing cancer treatment often means confronting a range of challenging side effects that can impact physical, emotional, and psychological well-being. From nausea and fatigue to hair loss and cognitive changes, these side effects can significantly disrupt daily life and pose additional hurdles on the path to recovery. However, with the right knowledge, strategies, and support, individuals can effectively manage and mitigate these side effects, empowering themselves to navigate the cancer journey with resilience and grace. Chemotherapy, radiation therapy, surgery, and other cancer treatments can trigger a variety of side effects that vary in severity and duration. Some of the most common side effects include:

- Nausea and vomiting.
- Fatigue.
- Hair loss.
- Changes in appetite.
- Pain.
- Cognitive difficulties (chemo brain).

- Emotional distress (anxiety, depression).

- Neuropathy (nerve damage).

- Skin changes.

- Mouth sores

By understanding the potential side effects associated with specific treatments, individuals can better prepare themselves and proactively address symptoms as they arise.

Nausea and vomiting are among the most dreaded side effects of cancer treatment, but there are several strategies available to help manage these symptoms. Anti-nausea medications, dietary modifications, acupuncture, and relaxation techniques can all provide relief and improve quality of life for patients undergoing chemotherapy or radiation therapy. It's essential to communicate openly with healthcare providers about the severity and frequency of nausea and vomiting to ensure appropriate management and support.

Fatigue is a common side effect experienced by cancer patients, often resulting from the physical and emotional toll of treatment. While rest is important, maintaining a balance between activity and rest can help prevent excessive fatigue and preserve energy levels. Gentle exercise, such as walking or yoga, can alleviate fatigue and improve overall well-being. Additionally, practicing good sleep hygiene, managing stress, and maintaining proper nutrition can support optimal energy levels throughout treatment.

Hair loss, changes in skin tone and texture, and weight fluctuations are common changes in appearance experienced by cancer patients undergoing treatment. While these changes can be emotionally challenging, there are ways to cope and maintain a sense of self-esteem and confidence. Wigs, scarves, and hats can provide temporary solutions for hair loss, while skincare products and makeup can help minimize the impact of skin changes. It's important for individuals to explore options that align with their preferences and comfort levels while navigating changes in appearance.

Many cancer patients experience cognitive changes, often referred to as "chemo brain," characterized by difficulties with memory, concentration, and multitasking. While these cognitive changes can be frustrating, there are strategies to help manage symptoms and improve cognitive function. Mindfulness practices, cognitive rehabilitation therapy, and memory aids such as calendars and to-do lists can all support cognitive functioning and enhance quality of life for individuals navigating chemo brain.

Emotional distress is a common side effect of cancer treatment, impacting individuals and their loved ones alike. Feelings of anxiety, depression, fear, and uncertainty are normal responses to a cancer diagnosis and can be exacerbated by treatment-related stressors. Seeking support from friends, family members, support groups, or mental health professionals can provide comfort, validation, and coping strategies for managing emotional challenges throughout the cancer journey.

Managing side effects is an integral aspect of the cancer experience, requiring patience, resilience, and adaptability from patients and their caregivers. By understanding common side effects, implementing proactive strategies, and seeking support from healthcare providers and loved ones, individuals can navigate treatment with greater ease and confidence. While side effects may present obstacles along the way, they also serve as reminders of the resilience and strength that reside within each person facing cancer. By embracing a holistic approach to symptom management and self-care, individuals can enhance their quality of life and cultivate a sense of empowerment in the face of adversity.q

Cancer survivorship has become an increasingly important aspect of cancer care, focusing on improving the quality of life for individuals who have completed treatment.

Chapter 14: Psychological Impact

The psychological impact of a cancer diagnosis extends far beyond the physical manifestations of the disease, profoundly influencing the emotional, social, and spiritual dimensions of a person's life. From the initial shock of diagnosis to the ongoing challenges of treatment and survivorship, individuals and their loved ones grapple with a complex array of emotions, ranging from fear and anxiety to hope and resilience. In this chapter, we explore the multifaceted psychological impact of cancer and provide insights, strategies, and support to help individuals navigate the emotional terrain with courage and grace.

A cancer diagnosis can trigger a whirlwind of emotions, including shock, disbelief, anger, sadness, and fear. These emotional responses are entirely normal reactions to a life-altering diagnosis and reflect the profound sense of uncertainty and vulnerability that accompanies the cancer journey. It's essential for individuals to acknowledge and validate their emotions, allowing themselves to grieve, express, and process their feelings in healthy and constructive ways.

Anxiety and fear are pervasive emotions experienced by many cancer patients, fueled by uncertainty about the future, concerns about treatment outcomes, and fear of recurrence. Learning to manage anxiety and fear requires cultivating coping mechanisms and support systems that provide comfort, reassurance, and a sense of control. Mindfulness practices, relaxation techniques, support groups, and therapy can all offer valuable tools for managing anxiety and fostering resilience in the face of uncertainty. Amidst the challenges of cancer, finding sources of hope and resilience can be a beacon of light in the darkness. Hope provides a sense of purpose, meaning, and optimism that sustains individuals through the darkest moments of their journey. Whether it's drawing strength from faith, connecting with supportive relationships, or finding inspiration in stories of survival, cultivating hope can empower individuals to face adversity with courage and determination.

A cancer diagnosis can profoundly impact a person's sense of identity and self-image, challenging long-held beliefs, roles, and expectations. Physical changes such as hair loss, weight fluctuations, and scars can alter one's perception of self, triggering feelings of insecurity, shame, and loss. It's important for individuals to acknowledge and accept these changes as part of their evolving journey, embracing self-compassion, self-care, and self-expression as they redefine their sense of identity and beauty.

Finding meaning and purpose in the midst of cancer can be a transformative and healing process, offering individuals a sense of agency, fulfillment, and connection amidst adversity. Engaging in activities that align with personal values, passions, and interests can provide a sense of purpose beyond the confines of illness, fostering a sense of vitality and vitality in the face of challenges. Whether it's pursuing creative outlets, volunteering, or advocating for causes dear to the heart, finding meaning in the cancer experience can empower individuals to reclaim agency and resilience in their lives. Navigating the psychological impact of cancer is not a journey to be undertaken alone.

Seeking support from loved ones, peers, support groups, and mental health professionals can provide invaluable comfort, validation, and guidance throughout the cancer journey. Sharing experiences, emotions, and challenges with others who understand can foster a sense of connection, belonging, and solidarity that eases the burden of illness and cultivates a sense of community and hope.

The psychological impact of cancer is profound and multifaceted, touching every aspect of a person's life and challenging them to confront their deepest fears, vulnerabilities, and strengths. By acknowledging and validating their emotions, cultivating resilience and hope, and seeking support from loved ones and professionals, individuals can navigate the emotional terrain of cancer with courage, grace, and resilience. While the journey may be fraught with challenges and uncertainties, it is also imbued with moments of profound growth, connection, and transformation that reaffirm the resilience of the human spirit in the face of adversity.

Chapter 15: Support Systems

In the face of a cancer diagnosis, the importance of support systems cannot be overstated. From family and friends to healthcare providers and community resources, a robust network of support plays a crucial role in empowering individuals to navigate the challenges of cancer with resilience, dignity, and hope. Personal relationships, including those with family members, friends, and caregivers, form the backbone of a cancer patient's support system. These individuals provide emotional support, practical assistance, and companionship during times of need, offering comfort, reassurance, and a sense of belonging amidst the challenges of illness. By fostering open communication, empathy, and trust within personal relationships, individuals can strengthen their support networks and enhance their ability to cope with the demands of cancer treatment and survivorship.

Healthcare providers, including oncologists, nurses, social workers, and other members of the healthcare team, play a pivotal role in supporting cancer patients throughout their journey. Building positive, collaborative relationships with healthcare providers fosters a sense of trust, partnership, and empowerment, enabling individuals to actively participate in their care and make informed decisions about treatment options and supportive services. Effective communication, advocacy, and shared decision-making are essential components of productive healthcare relationships that promote optimal outcomes and quality of life for cancer patients.

Support groups offer a unique forum for individuals affected by cancer to connect with others who share similar experiences, emotions, and challenges. Whether in-person or online, support groups provide a safe space for sharing stories, seeking advice, and offering mutual support and encouragement. Participating in support groups can reduce feelings of isolation, provide validation and understanding, and offer practical tips and resources for coping with the emotional and practical aspects of cancer. By engaging with support groups, individuals can cultivate a sense of community, belonging, and hope that strengthens their resilience and well-being throughout the cancer journey.

Community resources, such as cancer centers, nonprofit organizations, and advocacy groups, offer a wealth of support services and programs designed to meet the diverse needs of cancer patients and their families. These resources may include educational workshops, counseling services, financial assistance programs, transportation services, and peer mentorship programs, among others. By accessing community resources, individuals can supplement their existing support networks with additional services and resources that address specific needs and enhance their overall quality of life during and after cancer treatment.

In today's digital age, technology offers innovative ways to access support and connect with others affected by cancer. Online forums, social media groups, telehealth services, and mobile applications provide convenient platforms for sharing information, seeking support, and accessing resources from the comfort of home. By leveraging technology for support, individuals can overcome geographical barriers, connect with individuals from diverse backgrounds, and access a wealth of information and resources tailored to their unique needs and preferences.

While external support systems are invaluable, self-care practices also play a crucial role in supporting overall well-being during the cancer journey. Prioritizing self-care activities such as exercise, relaxation techniques, hobbies, and creative outlets can replenish physical, emotional, and spiritual reserves, reducing stress, enhancing resilience, and promoting a sense of balance and vitality amidst the challenges of cancer. By nurturing themselves, individuals can sustain their capacity to cope with adversity and thrive in the face of illness.

Support systems are essential lifelines that sustain individuals affected by cancer throughout their journey, offering comfort, strength, and hope in times of need. By cultivating and leveraging personal relationships, engaging with healthcare providers, accessing support groups and community resources, and embracing self-care practices, individuals can build robust networks of support that empower them to navigate the challenges of cancer with resilience, dignity, and grace. While the journey may be arduous and unpredictable, the presence of supportive relationships and resources serves as a beacon of light that illuminates the path forward, instilling courage, hope, and optimism in the face of adversity.

Genetic factors can also play a role in the development of cancer, with certain inherited mutations increasing an individual's risk.

Chapter 16: Survivorship

Survivorship marks the beginning of a new chapter in the cancer journey—a chapter defined by resilience, hope, and the pursuit of a fulfilling life beyond the confines of illness. As individuals transition from active treatment to life after cancer, they face a unique set of challenges and opportunities that shape their physical, emotional, and psychological well-being. Survivorship is more than just surviving; it's about thriving in the aftermath of cancer, reclaiming one's sense of self, and embracing life with renewed vitality and purpose. For many survivors, the transition from treatment to survivorship can be both liberating and daunting, marked by a mix of emotions ranging from relief and gratitude to anxiety and uncertainty. By acknowledging the challenges and opportunities of survivorship, individuals can cultivate a proactive mindset that empowers them to navigate the complexities of life after cancer with resilience and grace.

Physical and emotional health are central to survivorship, requiring ongoing attention, self-care, and support to promote optimal well-being. Regular follow-up care, including medical check-ups, screenings, and monitoring for late effects of treatment, is essential for detecting and addressing potential health issues early on. In addition to physical health, emotional well-being is equally important, as survivors may grapple with lingering feelings of fear, anxiety, depression, or post-traumatic stress related to their cancer experience. Seeking support from loved ones, healthcare providers, support groups, or mental health professionals can provide comfort, validation, and guidance for navigating the emotional challenges of survivorship.

While many cancer survivors experience relief and gratitude upon completing treatment, they may also face long-term side effects that impact their quality of life and daily functioning. These side effects may include fatigue, neuropathy, cognitive changes, lymphedema, sexual dysfunction, and others, depending on the type of cancer and treatments received. Managing long-term side effects requires a proactive approach, involving ongoing communication with healthcare providers, lifestyle modifications, and utilization of supportive therapies and resources tailored to individual needs.

Survivorship often prompts individuals to reflect on their sense of identity, purpose, and meaning in life, inviting them to redefine themselves beyond the label of "cancer survivor." This process of self-discovery and self-redefinition can be both liberating and challenging, as survivors navigate questions of identity, career, relationships, and life priorities in the wake of illness. Embracing survivorship as an opportunity for growth, self-expression, and personal fulfillment empowers individuals to cultivate a sense of purpose and resilience that transcends the limitations of their cancer experience.

Building connections and finding support within the survivorship community can be a source of strength, inspiration, and camaraderie for individuals navigating life after cancer. Support groups, survivorship programs, and peer mentorship initiatives offer valuable opportunities for survivors to share experiences, exchange advice, and forge meaningful connections with others who understand their journey. By engaging with the survivorship community, individuals can find validation, encouragement, and solidarity that enrich their survivorship experience and foster a sense of belonging and hope.

Celebrating milestones and achievements, both big and small, is an essential part of the survivorship journey, providing opportunities for reflection, gratitude, and resilience. Whether it's reaching a cancer-free milestone, returning to work or school, participating in a meaningful activity, or achieving a personal goal, each accomplishment signifies a triumph over adversity and a testament to the survivor's strength and resilience. By acknowledging and celebrating these milestones, survivors honor their journey, inspire others, and reaffirm their capacity to thrive in the face of challenges.

Survivorship is a journey of resilience, renewal, and possibility—a journey that extends far beyond the confines of illness and embraces the full spectrum of human experience. By embracing survivorship as an opportunity for growth, self-discovery, and personal fulfillment, individuals can reclaim their sense of agency, purpose, and vitality in the aftermath of cancer. With courage, optimism, and a supportive community by their side, survivors can navigate the challenges of survivorship with grace and resilience, embracing each new day as an opportunity to thrive and inspire others on their own survivorship journey.

Cancer survivorship has become an increasingly important aspect of cancer care, focusing on improving the quality of life for individuals who have completed treatment.

Chapter 17: Palliative Care

Palliative care is a holistic approach to supporting individuals facing serious illness, including cancer, by addressing their physical, emotional, and spiritual needs throughout the treatment process. Contrary to common misconceptions, palliative care is not synonymous with end-of-life care; rather, it focuses on enhancing quality of life, alleviating symptoms, and providing compassionate support for patients and their families at any stage of the illness. Palliative care is a specialized form of medical care that focuses on improving quality of life for individuals with serious illness, such as cancer, by addressing physical symptoms, managing pain, and providing holistic support for emotional, spiritual, and practical needs. Palliative care teams, comprised of healthcare professionals such as physicians, nurses, social workers, chaplains, and other specialists, work collaboratively to develop personalized care plans tailored to each patient's unique circumstances and preferences. By addressing the multidimensional needs of patients and their families, palliative care aims to enhance comfort, dignity, and overall well-being throughout the illness trajectory.

The benefits of palliative care extend beyond symptom management to encompass a range of physical, emotional, and practical advantages for patients and their families. Some of the key benefits of palliative care include:

- **Improved symptom management**: Palliative care teams specialize in alleviating symptoms such as pain, nausea, fatigue, and shortness of breath, enhancing comfort and quality of life for patients.

- **Enhanced communication and decision-making**: Palliative care providers facilitate open, honest discussions about treatment options, goals of care, and advance care planning, empowering patients and families to make informed decisions aligned with their values and preferences.

- **Emotional and spiritual support**: Palliative care addresses the emotional and spiritual needs of patients and families, providing counseling, spiritual care, and psychosocial support to navigate the challenges of serious illness with resilience and grace.

- **Coordination of care**: Palliative care teams collaborate with primary care providers, oncologists, specialists, and other healthcare professionals to ensure seamless coordination of care and support across different settings, optimizing continuity and quality of care for patients.

- **Support for caregivers**: Palliative care extends support to family caregivers, offering education, respite care, counseling, and practical assistance to alleviate caregiver burden and promote caregiver well-being.

Despite its many benefits, palliative care is often misunderstood and underutilized, with misconceptions about its scope, purpose, and timing prevailing among patients, families, and even healthcare providers. Some common misconceptions about palliative care include:

- **Palliative care is only for end-of-life**: Palliative care is appropriate for individuals at any stage of serious illness, regardless of prognosis or treatment goals. It focuses on enhancing quality of life and alleviating suffering, rather than prolonging life or hastening death.

- **Palliative care means giving up on treatment**: Palliative care is not mutually exclusive with curative treatment; rather, it complements and supports ongoing treatments such as chemotherapy, radiation therapy, and surgery. Palliative care providers work collaboratively with oncologists and other specialists to integrate symptom management and supportive care into the overall treatment plan.

- **Palliative care is only for physical symptoms**: While palliative care addresses physical symptoms, it also encompasses emotional, spiritual, and practical aspects of care, providing holistic support for patients and families facing serious illness.

- **Palliative care is only provided in hospice settings**: While palliative care is an essential component of hospice care for individuals nearing the end of life, it is also available in various settings, including hospitals, outpatient clinics, long-term care facilities, and even in patients' homes.

Integrating palliative care into cancer care can significantly enhance the quality of life and overall well-being of patients and their families. Early integration of palliative care, ideally at the time of diagnosis or early in the treatment process, allows patients to benefit from symptom management, psychosocial support, and advance care planning throughout their cancer journey. Palliative care providers collaborate closely with oncologists and other healthcare professionals to ensure comprehensive, patient-centered care that addresses the full spectrum of physical, emotional, and spiritual needs.

Palliative care represents a compassionate and holistic approach to supporting individuals and families facing serious illness, such as cancer, by addressing their physical, emotional, and spiritual needs with dignity and respect. By dispelling misconceptions, understanding the benefits, and integrating palliative care into cancer care early in the treatment process, individuals can experience enhanced comfort, quality of life, and overall well-being throughout the illness trajectory. As a vital component of comprehensive cancer care, palliative care serves as a beacon of hope and compassion, providing solace and support to patients and families on their journey through illness and beyond.

Chapter 18: End-of-Life Considerations

Navigating end-of-life considerations is perhaps one of the most challenging aspects of the cancer journey, requiring individuals and their loved ones to confront difficult decisions, emotions, and uncertainties with courage and compassion. As individuals face the reality of a terminal cancer diagnosis, it becomes essential to honor their personal values, beliefs, and preferences regarding end-of-life care. Advance care planning, including the completion of advance directives, living wills, and durable power of attorney for healthcare, allows individuals to express their wishes for medical treatment, life-sustaining measures, and end-of-life care in the event they are unable to communicate their preferences. By engaging in open, honest discussions with loved ones and healthcare providers, individuals can ensure their wishes are respected and upheld throughout the end-of-life journey.

Palliative care and hospice care play critical roles in supporting individuals and families facing terminal illness, offering comfort, symptom management, and emotional support during the end-of-life stage. Palliative care focuses on enhancing quality of life and relieving suffering for individuals with serious illness, regardless of prognosis or treatment goals. Hospice care, on the other hand, provides compassionate, interdisciplinary care for individuals with a prognosis of six months or less to live, emphasizing comfort and dignity in the final stages of life. By embracing palliative and hospice care, individuals can receive compassionate support and symptom management tailored to their unique needs and preferences, enabling them to live their remaining days with dignity and peace.

As individuals approach the end of life, they may face complex medical decisions regarding the use of life-sustaining treatments, resuscitation measures, and invasive procedures. These decisions can be emotionally challenging and fraught with uncertainty, requiring careful consideration of the benefits, burdens, and potential outcomes of various treatment options. Shared decision-making, facilitated by open communication between patients, families, and healthcare providers, allows individuals to make informed choices aligned with their values, goals, and preferences for end-of-life care. By engaging in thoughtful discussions and seeking guidance from trusted healthcare professionals, individuals can navigate complex medical decisions with clarity, compassion, and dignity.

End-of-life care encompasses not only physical comfort but also emotional and spiritual support for individuals and their families as they navigate the final stages of life. Social workers, chaplains, counselors, and other members of the healthcare team play crucial roles in providing compassionate support, counseling, and guidance to address the emotional, existential, and spiritual concerns of patients and families facing terminal illness. By fostering open communication, empathy, and compassionate presence, healthcare providers can create a supportive environment that honors the unique needs and beliefs of individuals and families during the end-of-life journey.

Despite the challenges and uncertainties of facing terminal illness, individuals and families can cultivate meaningful end-of-life experiences that honor life, love, and connection in the final stages of life. Creating opportunities for meaningful conversations, storytelling, reminiscence, and legacy-building allows individuals to reflect on their lives, express their love and gratitude, and leave a lasting impact on those they cherish. By embracing rituals, traditions, and activities that hold personal significance, individuals can create cherished memories and moments of connection that transcend the limitations of illness and bring comfort and solace to themselves and their loved ones.

As individuals approach the end of life, finding peace and closure becomes a central focus, allowing them to reconcile their lives, relationships, and legacies with a sense of acceptance and fulfillment. Spiritual practices, meditation, guided imagery, and other contemplative practices offer avenues for finding inner peace, comfort, and transcendence amidst the challenges of terminal illness. By embracing acceptance, letting go of regrets, and focusing on gratitude and love, individuals can approach the end of life with courage, grace, and dignity, finding solace in the knowledge that they have lived fully and loved deeply.

Navigating end-of-life considerations is a deeply personal and profound journey that requires courage, compassion, and support from individuals and their loved ones. By honoring personal values and preferences, embracing palliative and hospice care, navigating complex medical decisions, providing emotional and spiritual support, cultivating meaningful end-of-life experiences, and finding peace and closure, individuals can approach the end of life with dignity, comfort, and grace. As we journey through the final stages of life, may we find solace in the love, connections, and memories that sustain us, and may we embrace each moment with gratitude, acceptance, and peace.

Cancer prevention efforts also include vaccination against certain viruses that can cause cancer, such as human papillomavirus (HPV) and hepatitis B virus (HBV).

Chapter 19: Advances in Research

The landscape of cancer research is continually evolving, driven by relentless scientific inquiry, technological advancements, and collaborative efforts aimed at unraveling the complexities of the disease and improving outcomes for patients worldwide. Recent years have witnessed unprecedented advancements in our understanding of the molecular underpinnings of cancer, fueled by breakthroughs in genomics, proteomics, and molecular biology. High-throughput sequencing technologies, such as next-generation sequencing (NGS), have enabled researchers to decipher the genetic alterations, mutations, and molecular pathways driving cancer initiation, progression, and resistance to therapy. These insights have paved the way for the development of targeted therapies, precision medicine approaches, and personalized treatment strategies tailored to the unique genetic profiles of individual patients.

Immunotherapy has emerged as a transformative approach to cancer treatment, harnessing the power of the immune system to recognize, attack, and eliminate cancer cells. Checkpoint inhibitors, chimeric antigen receptor (CAR) T-cell therapy, cancer vaccines, and adoptive cell transfer are among the innovative immunotherapeutic strategies revolutionizing the field of oncology. By unleashing the body's immune response against cancer, immunotherapy offers durable responses, improved survival outcomes, and the potential for long-term remission in a variety of cancer types, including melanoma, lung cancer, and hematologic malignancies.

In addition to traditional cytotoxic chemotherapy and targeted therapies, researchers are exploring novel therapeutic modalities that hold promise for the treatment of cancer. These include oncolytic viruses, gene editing technologies such as CRISPR-Cas9, RNA interference (RNAi) therapies, and epigenetic modifiers that target aberrant gene expression in cancer cells. By leveraging innovative approaches and cutting-edge technologies, researchers aim to overcome treatment resistance, enhance therapeutic efficacy, and minimize off-target effects, ushering in a new era of precision oncology and personalized medicine.

Early detection and screening are critical components of cancer prevention and management, enabling the timely diagnosis and intervention of cancer at its earliest, most treatable stages. Advances in imaging technologies, liquid biopsy techniques, and biomarker discovery have facilitated the development of non-invasive, high-sensitivity screening tests for various cancer types, including breast, colorectal, prostate, and lung cancer. By detecting cancer earlier, researchers aim to improve survival rates, reduce treatment morbidity, and enhance overall outcomes for patients.

Artificial intelligence (AI) and machine learning algorithms are revolutionizing cancer research and clinical practice, offering powerful tools for data analysis, pattern recognition, and predictive modeling. By mining vast repositories of clinical, genomic, and imaging data, AI-driven approaches can identify novel biomarkers, predict treatment response, and optimize treatment strategies tailored to individual patient characteristics. Furthermore, AI-powered diagnostic tools, decision support systems, and digital health technologies are transforming cancer care delivery, enhancing efficiency, accuracy, and accessibility for patients and providers alike.

Collaboration and knowledge-sharing are essential drivers of progress in cancer research, fostering interdisciplinary partnerships and collective efforts to tackle the most pressing challenges in oncology. Initiatives such as The Cancer Genome Atlas (TCGA), the Precision Medicine Initiative, and international consortia bring together researchers, clinicians, industry partners, and patient advocates to accelerate the pace of discovery, translation, and implementation of innovative cancer therapies and technologies. By fostering a culture of collaboration and open science, these initiatives aim to maximize the impact of cancer research and improve outcomes for patients worldwide.

The landscape of cancer research is characterized by unprecedented innovation, collaboration, and progress, driven by the collective efforts of scientists, clinicians, patients, and advocates worldwide. From unraveling the molecular complexities of cancer to harnessing the power of the immune system and leveraging cutting-edge technologies, advances in research are transforming the future of cancer care and survivorship. As we continue to push the boundaries of knowledge and innovation, may we remain steadfast in our commitment to advancing science, improving outcomes, and ultimately conquering cancer for the benefit of all those affected by the disease.

Lifestyle factors such as maintaining a healthy weight, eating a balanced diet, exercising regularly, avoiding tobacco, limiting alcohol consumption, and practicing sun safety can help reduce the risk of developing cancer.

Chapter 20: The Role of Technology

In the modern era, technology has become an indispensable ally in the fight against cancer, revolutionizing every aspect of prevention, diagnosis, treatment, and survivorship. From cutting-edge imaging techniques and genomic sequencing technologies to artificial intelligence-driven diagnostics and telemedicine platforms, technological innovations have transformed the landscape of cancer care, offering new possibilities for improved outcomes, enhanced patient experiences, and personalized approaches to treatment. Advancements in imaging technologies have revolutionized the early detection, diagnosis, and staging of cancer, enabling clinicians to visualize tumors with unprecedented precision and accuracy. Techniques such as magnetic resonance imaging (MRI), positron emission tomography (PET), computed tomography (CT), and molecular imaging modalities provide detailed insights into tumor morphology, metabolism, and molecular characteristics, guiding treatment decisions and monitoring response to therapy. Furthermore, emerging technologies such as optical coherence tomography (OCT), photoacoustic imaging, and multiparametric imaging hold promise for further enhancing diagnostic capabilities and improving patient outcomes.

The advent of genomic sequencing technologies has ushered in a new era of precision medicine, enabling researchers and clinicians to unravel the molecular complexities of cancer and tailor treatment strategies to individual patient characteristics. Next-generation sequencing (NGS), whole genome sequencing (WGS), and RNA sequencing (RNA-seq) technologies facilitate comprehensive genomic profiling of tumors, identifying genetic alterations, mutations, and biomarkers that drive cancer initiation, progression, and treatment response. By integrating genomic data with clinical information, researchers can develop targeted therapies, immunotherapies, and combination treatment approaches that maximize therapeutic efficacy while minimizing toxicity and treatment resistance.

Artificial intelligence (AI) and machine learning algorithms are revolutionizing cancer research and clinical practice, offering powerful tools for data analysis, pattern recognition, and predictive modeling. AI-driven approaches enable researchers to identify novel biomarkers, predict treatment response, and optimize treatment strategies tailored to individual patient characteristics. Furthermore, AI-powered diagnostic tools, decision support systems, and digital health technologies are transforming cancer care delivery, enhancing efficiency, accuracy, and accessibility for patients and providers alike.

Telemedicine platforms and remote monitoring technologies have emerged as valuable tools for expanding access to cancer care, particularly in underserved communities and rural areas. Telehealth consultations, virtual tumor boards, and remote monitoring devices enable patients to receive timely medical advice, follow-up care, and supportive services from the comfort of their homes, reducing the burden of travel and improving convenience and accessibility. Furthermore, telemedicine facilitates multidisciplinary collaboration among healthcare providers, enabling seamless coordination of care and support across different settings.

Digital health technologies empower patients to actively participate in their care and make informed decisions about their health and well-being. Mobile applications, wearable devices, and patient portals enable individuals to track symptoms, monitor treatment side effects, access educational resources, and communicate with healthcare providers in real-time. By fostering patient engagement, self-management, and shared decision-making, digital health technologies enhance patient-centered care and promote empowerment, autonomy, and resilience in the face of cancer.

While technology holds immense promise for advancing cancer care and improving patient outcomes, it also presents challenges and ethical considerations that must be addressed. These include issues related to data privacy and security, interoperability of electronic health records, disparities in access to technology, and concerns about over-reliance on automation and algorithmic decision-making. Furthermore, the rapid pace of technological innovation requires ongoing education, training, and evaluation to ensure that healthcare providers and patients alike can harness the full potential of technology in a safe, effective, and ethical manner.

Technology has become an indispensable ally in the fight against cancer, transforming every aspect of the cancer journey from prevention and diagnosis to treatment and survivorship. By harnessing the power of imaging and diagnostics, genomic and precision medicine, artificial intelligence and machine learning, telemedicine and remote monitoring, and digital health technologies, researchers and clinicians are revolutionizing cancer care and improving outcomes for patients worldwide. As we continue to innovate and adapt to the evolving landscape of technology, may we remain steadfast in our commitment to harnessing the full potential of technology to conquer cancer and improve the lives of those affected by the disease.

The early stages of cancer may not produce noticeable symptoms, which is why regular screenings and early detection are crucial for improving outcomes.

Chapter 21: Global Efforts in Cancer Control

Cancer is a global health challenge that transcends borders, affecting individuals, families, and communities worldwide. Recognizing the urgent need to address the burden of cancer and improve access to prevention, early detection, treatment, and palliative care services, governments, international organizations, healthcare professionals, researchers, and advocates have mobilized efforts to develop comprehensive cancer control strategies and initiatives. Cancer represents one of the leading causes of morbidity and mortality worldwide, accounting for millions of deaths annually and imposing a significant economic and social burden on individuals, families, and societies. The burden of cancer is disproportionately borne by low- and middle-income countries (LMICs), where access to cancer prevention, diagnosis, and treatment services is often limited due to systemic barriers, resource constraints, and disparities in healthcare infrastructure and financing. Addressing the global burden of cancer requires a coordinated, multisectoral approach that prioritizes equity, access, and sustainability in cancer control efforts.

The World Health Organization (WHO) plays a central role in coordinating global efforts to address the burden of cancer and promote cancer prevention, early detection, treatment, and palliative care services worldwide. Through initiatives such as the Global Initiative for Cancer Registry Development (GICR), the International Agency for Research on Cancer (IARC), and the World Cancer Report, the WHO provides technical assistance, capacity-building support, and evidence-based guidance to countries in developing and implementing national cancer control plans and strategies. Furthermore, the WHO collaborates with governments, civil society organizations, and other stakeholders to advocate for policy changes, resource mobilization, and investments in cancer prevention and control.

Many countries have developed national cancer control plans (NCCPs) to guide their efforts in addressing the burden of cancer and improving access to comprehensive cancer care services for their populations. NCCPs typically encompass a range of strategies and interventions aimed at cancer prevention, early detection, diagnosis, treatment, and palliative care, as well as efforts to address cancer risk factors, reduce disparities, and strengthen health systems. By adopting a systematic, evidence-based approach to cancer control, countries can optimize resource allocation, prioritize interventions, and maximize the impact of their efforts in reducing the burden of cancer and improving outcomes for patients.

Effective cancer control requires collaboration and partnerships across multiple sectors, including government, healthcare, academia, industry, civil society, and the community. Multisectoral collaboration facilitates knowledge-sharing, resource mobilization, and coordinated action to address the complex interplay of factors contributing to the burden of cancer, including social determinants of health, environmental exposures, and lifestyle behaviors. Through initiatives such as the United Nations Sustainable Development Goals (SDGs), the

Global Cancer Observatory (GCO), and the World Cancer Leaders' Summit, stakeholders come together to exchange best practices, advocate for policy changes, and mobilize resources to accelerate progress in cancer control globally.

Disparities in access to cancer care services persist both within and between countries, exacerbating the burden of cancer and undermining efforts to achieve equitable health outcomes for all. Addressing disparities requires a multifaceted approach that addresses social, economic, and structural barriers to care, including poverty, lack of education, inadequate healthcare infrastructure, and limited access to essential medicines and technologies. By prioritizing equity, access, and inclusivity in cancer control efforts, stakeholders can ensure that all individuals, regardless of socioeconomic status, geography, or other factors, have access to timely, affordable, and high-quality cancer care services.

Research and innovation are fundamental drivers of progress in cancer control, enabling the development of new prevention strategies, diagnostic tools, treatment modalities, and supportive care interventions. By investing in research and innovation, countries can accelerate the pace of discovery, translation, and implementation of evidence-based interventions that improve outcomes for cancer patients and reduce the burden of the disease. Collaborative research networks, funding initiatives, and knowledge-sharing platforms facilitate global cooperation and coordination in cancer research, fostering a culture of innovation and excellence in the fight against cancer.

Global efforts in cancer control represent a shared commitment to addressing the burden of cancer and improving outcomes for individuals and communities worldwide. By prioritizing equity, access, and sustainability in cancer control efforts, stakeholders can overcome systemic barriers, reduce disparities, and ensure that all individuals have access to timely, affordable, and high-quality cancer care services. Through collaboration, innovation, and advocacy, we can harness the collective power of the global community to confront the challenges of cancer and build a future where cancer is no longer a barrier to health, dignity, and well-being for all.

Special Bonus

Gain access to all my previous and future books

Please consider writing a review!